THE ORIGINAL #2020 KETO DIET SLOW COOKER RECIPE BOOK

Quick and Healthy Keto Diet Recipes for Your Slow Cooker incl. 14 Days Weight Loss Plan

Catherine J. Emsworth

ISBN- 9798663373531

TABLE OF CONTENTS

TABLE OF CONTENTS

5

THE MEANING OF KETOGENIC

The ketogenic diet is becoming more popular amongst those who want to follow a healthy eating plan. This type of healthy eating is championed by many famous people and celebrities but what exactly is ketogenic?

Is the Keto Diet for you?

The Ketogenic Diet is often known as the keto diet, and it is the process of eating low-carb, high-fat (LCHF) foods. By doing this, you restrict carbohydrates which in turn deprives your body of glucose sugars which the body uses for energy. When you do not have enough glucose in your body to burn, your body looks to another way of gaining energy, and as a result your body will burn fat stores. This in turn sees your body producing ketones in your liver to get the energy that you need, and the body goes into a state of ketosis.

Therefore, the best way to explain ketosis is how your body breaks stored fats to provide energy by producing ketones. The ketogenic diet is made up of 75% healthy fats, 20% protein and 5% carbohydrates.

Controlling your metabolism with Keto Diet

According to those already following this type of eating the Keto diet reprograms your metabolism. It is the metabolic system that provides your body with the energy needed to function. When your body is in nutritional ketosis you are burning fats whilst eating healthy fats, which means that you are boosting your metabolism.

Starving and severely reducing calories in your diet see your metabolic rate fall and this can be dangerous for your metabolism, but this is not the way a keto diet works, as it increases your metabolism to continually burn fat. For this reason, following a diet that is low in carbohydrates alone will not work as the body still requires a source of fuel and therefore, providing your body with healthy fats to burn is how you can keep stable control of your metabolism.

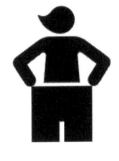

HOW DOES KETOGENIC WORK WITH WEIGHT LOSS?

If you starve yourself or reduce your calorie intake you will lose weight, however, your metabolism will also drop, and this is what leads to plateaus and you will gain the weight you have lost over again.

When you put your body into ketosis, you are not lowering your calories necessarily, but you are consuming low levels of carbohydrates with moderate portions of protein and a high proportion of fat. The process of keto also has a diuretic effect on your body therefore, when you begin the diet you will drop pounds immediately due to water weight loss. It is important that you provide your body with electrolytes and this is achieved by drinking lots of water as your body is adjusting and becoming a fat burning vessel.

Once your metabolic rate increases you will be surprised by the amount of weight you can lose even though you are still having high-fat foods such as butter, cheese, bacon and beef in your diet.

The keto diet was originally described as a method that prevented children having epileptic fits, yet the keto diet has been used since for a multitude of reasons.

Restricting carbohydrates and filling your body with high fats will drive your body to burn the fat that it has stored and produce ketones, and it is these ketones that can then be used as your energy source. Increased levels of ketones on your blood is beneficial to your health.

As well as weight loss you will find that following a strict keto diet will lead to improvements to your immune system, an increased metabolic rate, less inflammation in your body, the reversal of any types of cognitive impairments, controlled blood sugars, lowered risk of cancer, a clearer mind, a reduction in the risk of cardiovascular disease, an improvement in your skin, higher levels of HDL cholesterol which is the good cholesterol, a reduced risk of suffering from Type 2 diabetes and improved levels of triglyceride.

As with every benefit there are usually some sort of side effects and those that have been reported are craving carbohydrates, fatigue, irritability, constipation and sleeping problems. If you do find that you suffer from any of the above, you can modify your diet and increase carbs if you wish. It is just a case of finding out what works for you until you have reached your goal and can maintain the weight you want to be.

Eventually, anyone in ketosis will not only feel better but they will also find that they can perform better. Even though the body fat will drop dramatically your vitality and energy will improve. Most people that master and are successful following a ketogenic eating plan do not see it as a diet or healthy eating regime, they see it as a lifestyle.

WORKING TOWARDS A KETO DIET

The ketogenic diet has been popular and only really heard about for the past few years. You may have read about the ketogenic diet in a magazine or maybe a friend or work colleague is following it and you find yourself wondering why and how it works.

The mainstream media along with nutritionists and dietitians have drummed it into people that all types of fat is bad for you and should be reduced in your diet. By reporting that the way to go is high-carb, low-fat if you want to lead a healthy life, preaching that high-fat diets will lead to increased blood pressure and cholesterol levels, as well as heart disease and other types of health-related issues. However, studies have shown that this is not the case and that eating a diet that is low in carbohydrates and high in fat can provide you with many health benefits. In this book I will introduce you to ketogenic eating, how your health can be improved which are shown above plus how you can lose weight using the keto diet plan, also how you can tell if you have reached a ketogenic state.

The ketogenic diet works on the principles of high-fat and low-carb, with the aim of entering ketosis which sees you burning ketones instead of where your body is burning ketones instead of glucose as its energy source. I hear you saying, "How does this way of eating work, and how can I get myself into a ketogenic state? Keep reading to find out more.

Peoples diets have only changed in the last ten years with most eating a carbohydrate rich diet with some protein and a minimal amount of fat. If you eat a meal that is rich in carbohydrate your body turns the carbs to glucose and your body can then use them for its energy source.

This is where the ketogenic diet turns the diet around, carbohydrates are eaten in small amounts and this is what will force your body to use another source of energy. As there are no carbohydrates as such to convert the body needs to get the energy from another source to maintain its functions. When there are no carbohydrates your liver takes the fatty acids and transforms these into ketones as its energy source. This state is known as ketosis and what everyone following a ketogenic diet strives to get to.

When your body breaks down the fatty acids, they divide into three types of ketones the first is Acetoacetate (AcAc), next is acetone and finally Beta-hydroxybutyric acid (BHB) which is a combination of the first two ketones.

What can you eat on a Keto Diet?

When you follow a keto diet, you need to be aware that you will have to eat a huge amount of fat, as the majority calories will come from the fat you consume, in conjunction with the protein and tiny carbohydrates.

The keto diet works through a process that is macronutrient breakdown. People who are already eating a low carb diet could have to eat even less to get them to healthy ketosis. When following a keto menu, you will have to eat foods such as olive oil, nuts, seeds, avocado and other high fat foods, you also need to include eggs, seafood, quality meat and full fat dairy.

Your fiber will come from the minerals and vitamins that are in leafy green vegetables such as spinach, cauliflower, Brussels sprouts and so on.

When you are following a keto plan, you need to steer clear of grains even wholegrain as well as sugar and starch. Ideally your diet should have not more than 30 grams of carbohydrates a day.

Finally it is vital that you do not restrict the number of calories you are consuming on a keto diet as this will see you not eating enough particularly as you have cut out sugar and carbs, your body still needs the energy to function properly.

Unlimited Protein

You may think that you should not consume much protein whilst following a keto diet, but this is not so as it will not affect your ability to get to ketosis.

Everyone has gluconeogenesis (GNG), and this process is usually misunderstood but is a metabolic process. There are some that say that if you eat large amounts of protein GNG becomes active and our blood sugar increases, this is not true.

The truth is that GNG makes glucose from all non-carbohydrates and includes lactate, protein and glycerol and this is the usual process that is vital to fuel the tissues in the body that cannot use ketones such as your red blood cells, certain parts of the brain and testicles.

Maintaining levels of Blood glucose

It is important for you to build glycogen as without this ketosis is not possible, ketones are an exceptional source of fuel, but they cannot fuel every bodily process, and this is when GNG steps in and fuels everything else. GNG is a stable commodity therefore if you were to eat more protein than a standard keto diet allows your GNG will not force your body from its ketogenic state.

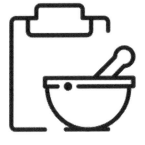

DIFFERENT KETO DIETS

You may be surprised but there are four different types of keto diet, these are the standard, targeted, cyclical and high protein. Each approach will help you to burn fat, lose weight and stabilize your blood sugars however they all provide you with different objectives and benefits.

We will now look at the different keto diet plans, the Target Keto diet (TKD) is for those who work out for hours and endurance athletes.

Standard Keto Diet

This is the most common type of keto diet and is ideal for beginners and those wanting to lose body fat and for those who are insulin resistant.

On this form of keto plan, you would be consuming a good amount of protein, about 0.8g of protein per pound of body mass. 20 – 50 g of net carbs or 5% of your calorie intake and 70 – 75% of your total calorie intake should come from fat.

High Protein Keto Diet

This is very similar to the Standard Keto Diet although you eat more protein, the extra protein is needed to build muscle. In this diet the aim is to get your calories in the following quantities, 60% from fat, 35% from protein and 5% from carbohydrates. This is a popular type of Keto particularly with people that need more protein in their diet.

Cyclical Keto Diet

The CKD (cyclical keto) sees you eating low carbs which are then followed by keto for the next few days then a couple of days eating a diet that is high in carbohydrates. On this diet you move through two diet phases a standard keto diet follows by a carbohydrate loaded diet. The high carbohydrate phase can last from 24 – 48 hours and you will get approximately 70% of your calories from carbs. A week on this plan would be as follows:

Day 1 – 5: Your calories will be distributed as fat 70% - 75%, protein 20% - 25%, carbs 5%

Day 6 & 7: Carb loading where your calories will be split as carbohydrates 70%, protein 20 – 25% and fat 10 – 15%

This eating plan is ideal for athletes to assist with maximize fat loss and build lean muscle.

Targeted Keto Diet

As you are now au fait with the three different ways you can undertake the keto eating plan, we will now look at the TKD which targets the amount of carbohydrates you consume based on your workouts. TKD is ideal to maintain exercise performance whilst fuelling your muscles during exercise.

If you decide you wish to give this a go you should consume 25 – 50g of net carbohydrates and ½ - 1 hour before you exercise, and this equates to your carbohydrates for the day.

This type of diet is a combination of the cyclical and standard ketogenic diet. It provides you with what your body needs to train harder and does not force your body out of ketosis for any long period of time.

YOU AND THE TARGETED KETOGENIC DIET

There is no knowing which keto diet you will get on with and knowing which will provide you with the fastest fat loss. However, if you are new to keto it would probably be a good idea to start with the standard keto diet, and if you find that your athletic performance drops off switch to the TKD to see the difference in the results. You need to be mindful that you need to eat enough carbohydrates to supply your muscles with enough glycogen.

How to Become Fat Adapted

The state of ketosis is a natural function. If your body was to undergo long periods without food, it would fall into ketosis. Many of us enter ketosis first thing in the morning as our bodies have gone for 10 – 12 hours without food. The people who are in keto are in effect starving their body if carbohydrates so that it must turn to the fat for energy.

When your body first runs on ketones you may find that you experience some effects which could include feeling as though you have the flu, feeling lethargic, headaches and mild sickness. However, sticking with it will see your body preferring to use fat for energy as it adapts to keto. You then should find out if the keto diet is working for you and whether you can stay in ketosis and you can only find out about this if you check the level of ketones in your body.

Making sure you are in Ketosis

The only way that you will know whether you have got into and stayed in ketosis is to test the ketone levels in your body. It is important to test the levels to ensure that you are getting the full benefits that this type of diet can give you.

As soon as your body begins to burn fat for fuel you enter ketosis and the blood ketones spill into your breath, blood and urine, and this is how you can test them.

Breath test

The ketone that shows up on your breath is known as acetone and this can be tested using a breath meter, unfortunately this is not the most reliable and therefore you should not use it as your only testing method.

Blood Test

The most accurate and reliable way to monitor your ketone level is by a blood test. You can use a blood glucose meter with blood strip and the only downside is that this can be rather expensive particularly if you test frequently.

Urine Testing

It is easy to buy urine strips and then work out the level of ketone by colour. The problem with this test is that it is not always reliable particularly if you have reached and stayed in ketosis for a sometime as your electrolyte and hydration levels can also affect the reason.

KETO-ADAPTATION

The Keto-adaptation also referred to as fat-adaptation and this is the process your body undergoes when it uses fat instead of glucose for energy. Ketones are water molecules that come from the liver when it metabolizes fats especially when the intake of carbohydrates are low. Ketones can be used by most areas of the body which are unable to use unrefined fats for its fuel.

The word "keto" is the shortened name given to ketones, and these are molecules that are water-soluble created by the liver makes when metabolizing fats, especially when you are only eating small amounts of carbohydrates.

Our bodies continually use a mixture of glucose and fat for energy; however, this is when they are in a non keto state. The body reaches for the glucose first as there are only small amounts of ketones that can be constructed through the metabolization of fat. Some of the tissues such as the heart prefers to use ketones when it can, and the brain cannot use fat therefore it is dependent on glucose when the body is in a non-keto state.

Your Keto State

When your sources of glucose run out your brain and various organs begin to adapt and use fats and the ketones instead of glucose as the main fuel. But getting into ketosis where the fats and ketones are providing your body with its fuel is not a nice experience.

To start with the extremely restrictive carbohydrate can lead to adverse side effects such as fatigue, nausea and weakness. Although it takes everyone their own amount of time to adapt to keto the process usually starts within the first few days. After the first week people will usually feel the positive effects with reports which have included improved concentration and more energy. Once you get to the end of week two, although this can be three weeks for some the body has accomplished most of the work needed to get its energy from fat. Any food cravings or hunger pangs with have gone and your vitality and stamina are increased.

The body then keeps making subtle changes such as conserving protein so the cravings for protein are diminished. Many athletes have noticed that there is less lactic acid build up when they have done longer training sessions in the terms of soreness and fatigue. It is worth remembering that it can take a while for your body to change and keto to be fully reached.

Adapt Your Body

There are various ways to get through the first week when you have withdrawn carbohydrate from your diet, but the best advice I can give is to eat plenty of fiber and plenty of fat as feeling full will see you missing your carbs less. ou should also make a concentrated effort to increase both your water and salt intake. Once of the side effects following a keto plan is that you lose fluids and electrolytes. Carbohydrates hold water and therefore cutting them out of your diet will see you necding to drink more to replenish your body. It is also advisable to ease yourself into your exercise plans start with walking and stretching for the first few weeks.

THE ADVANTAGES AND DISADVANTAGES OF KETO

Advantages

Weight Loss

Your body goes into fat burning mode when it enters ketosis, and this supports fat loss. By cutting carbohydrates your body retains less water and this also contributes towards weight loss. As carbohydrates have fewer calories the body digests them quicker which makes you blood glucose spike then crash again and they are not that satisfying, granted you feel full for a while after eating but you also feel hungry so much more quickly that if you had eaten fats or proteins.

Fats are so much more satisfying that when people switch and start a low carbohydrate diet and replace their carbs with fats, they will that they cannot eat as much therefore their calorie intake is decreased leading to weight loss.

Enhanced Satisfaction and Reduced Appetite

You already know that you can expect to lose weight on a keto diet as you will eat less. The high fat content that is in the keto plan reduces carbohydrate cravings as the high fat provides you with a steady supply of energy.

Lower Cholesterol

It may seem unbelievable that you can eat fat and reduce your cholesterol, but it is true. Well to a certain degree, the cholesterol you should be concerned with. Research has shown that a keto diet can improve "good cholesterol" known as HDL and lower the "bad cholesterol" known as LDL. The higher your HDL levels the lower your risk of heart complications.

Lower Risk of Heart Disease

It is true that fat has been long thought of as bad and unhealthy and carbohydrates and grains were good for you. However, research into this has shown that reducing the amount of carbohydrates in your diet can reduce your blood triglycerides, which are fat molecules found in your blood. Having higher levels puts you at a greater risk regarding heart disease.

Lower Your Blood Pressure

Studies have confirmed that by eating a diet that is low in carbohydrates has positive impact on blood pressure. High blood pressure (Hypertension) is a risk for various diseases including kidney failure, heart disease and stroke,

Insulin Level Reduction and Resistance

It has been proven that following a keto diet can reduce insulin spikes and reduce blood sugars because of the reduced consumption of carbohydrates. Having better control of your insulin can also improve any symptoms or metabolic disorders that are due to high blood sugars and insulin.

Improvement in Cognitive Function

The improvement in cognitive function is possibly the best perk of adapting a keto diet. Fat converts to ketones in the liver and this is then sent to the brain, ketones can cross the barrier of the blood and brain to be used as energy for the brain cells.

Epilepsy in children has been treated for years using the keto diet and studies are currently underway to see the potential in come play in neurological diseases.

Enhanced Sleep, Energy and Mood

Many people profess to needing more sleep however this is not the benefit a ketogenic diet offers, as many people that follow a ketogenic diet find that they need less sleep when in ketosis. They feel more energetic and alert on the same amount of sleep.

As the hormones are no longer dealing with insulin highs and lows most people find that they feel more stable and as such find themselves in a far better mood.

Boost your Energy

Eating a meal that is carb heavy will probably make you feel lethargic and even sleepy, this is because your insulin has spiked and your blood sugars dropper. By eating a diet that is high in fat your body is provided with steady energy and this helps to avoid the crashes sustained when eating a high carbohydrate diet. Also due to the brain preferring ketones for its source of energy the high fat diet will leave you feeling far more energized without the need to supply a steady influx of calories.

Regulated Hormones

Apart from weight loss, one of the main reason's women are so eager to follow a keto diet is the hormone balance. Women that suffer from imbalanced hormones could gain relief from a keto diet and research has shown that the keto diet can assist with infertility issues as well as longevity and thyroid health.

Disadvantages

As we have seen above there are plenty of advantages of keto, however there are also some disadvantages that you do need to consider.

The Adaptation Process

To become keto adapted can be a difficult road for some and this can take 1 – 2 weeks. You may experience flu like symptoms during your transition period which include but are not limited to fatigue, headaches, nausea and general malaise.

A loss of electrolytes is possible as your body is not going to retain as much water because of the restricted carbohydrates. This is easy to fix by taking a mineral supplement.

Intestinal Problems

As you are increasing the fat in your diet and reducing your carbohydrate may see you suffering from constipation or diarrhoea. Once your body becomes fat-adapted this should resolve itself. You could also suffer with nausea when you switch from a low-fat to a keto diet. The liver, gall bladder and pancreas can take a while to adapt to digesting large amounts of fat.

Certain Foods are Restricted

There are some people that are not in agreeance with banning an entire food group. The keto diet means you will have to give up all types of sugar as well as popular forms of carbohydrates such as pasta, bread, burgers, pizzas and so on.

Most fruits are also limited due to their fructose content and starch vegetables such as corn and potatoes. The only good thing is that once your body is adapted the sugar carvings will reduce dramatically or go away altogether.

High Cholesterol

Generally, most people see their weight and cholesterol levels fall, however there are some people that could see the opposite due to the heavy meat content of this diet. This is a genetic vulnerability and does prove that the keto diet is not for everyone.

Harder for Entertaining

It can be difficult to eat out or attend social gatherings as you will need to plan and even research to ensure that you will be able to stick to your keto diet. The key here is to be more self-disciplined. When it comes to alcohol you should limit yourself to one of two drinks that are low in carbohydrates. This means the driest wine or clear liquid such as gin, vodka etc.

WHAT CAN YOU EAT?

If you have thought about giving a new diet a go to lose some weight the keto diet may have sprung to mind. Due to celebrities such as Halle Berry and Kourtney Kardashian endorsing this way of living the Keto diet has been pushed to the front of any diet plans. Anyway, there are few diets where you can still eat vast amounts of cheese and bacon!

Whilst I could list the things that ou can or cannot eat you still need to know how it works. The main principles of this diet are to maintain ketosis. This is the metabolic rate that pushes your body to burn fat for its fuel rather than the glucose it can get from carbohydrates.

This way of eating was originally developed to help people combat epilepsy and a keto diet is meant to guide you into ketosis by removing some significant groups of foods that you would normally use on a daily basis such as foods that contain sugars and carbohydrates, because these so not allow your metabolism to use fat as its main energy source.

Whilst may not think that sugar and Carbohydrates have a place in a healthy meal, they are found in nutritious items that you are going to have to exclude from your diet. For this reason, health experts' and nutritionists may appear critical of keto as strong will power is required to make sure you are excluding the required elements. It is true that keto can see serious weight loss for those who stick with it, but the keto diet is not for everyone particularly those who know they cannot give up fruit or bread. Something more flexible such as the Mediterranean diet is more flexible and could help with weight loss goals.

Even if you have seen the amazing transformation some people have undergone whilst following a ketogenic diet, I urge you to read about keto so that you are well informed about everything before you try to achieve ketosis. In the same way as many diets the keto way of eating does not guarantee that you will maintain the weight loss and for this reason you need to speak to your doctor or healthcare provider before making any long-term changes to your diet.

Keto Diet Foods

When it comes to what you can eat when following a keto diet, you need to prepare yourself for a vast amount of fat, some protein and no carbohydrates through your day. Get ready for a whole lot of fat, some protein, and just about zero carbs throughout your day. Your fridge and or pantry should contain lots of meat, dairy, seafood, fats, eggs, oil and any vegetables that grow above ground.

You can eat plenty of chicken, steak, lamb, pork, turkey, ham, bacon, ground beef and small quantities of sausage.

Seafood including snapper, halibut, cod, scallops, catfish, salmon and trout, as well as shellfish such as clams, oysters, mussels and lobster.

Oils and most fats including mayonnaise, butter, coconut and olive oil, ghee, avocados and avocado oil, lard and eggs.

Dairy with a high-fat content such as soft and hard cheeses, sour cream, cream cheese and heavy cream.

Certain vegetables including cabbage, cauliflower, zucchini, broccoli, peppers, onion, cucumber, eggplant, tomatoes, green beans, asparagus, spinach, lettuce, mushroom, lettuce, and olives.

Most nuts and nut butters but be sure to look for natural buttes that do not include any sweetener.

Berries such as raspberries, blueberries and blackberries.

Various drinks such as unsweetened coffee and black tea. Champagne, dry wine and spirits can be drunk but very sparingly.

You can also enjoy sucralose and stevia occasionally.

Foods that you must avoid when you are following a keto diet will probably include many of your favourites and the list is endless. In simple terms you need to avoid most starches and sugars as well as pasta, rice, bread, corn, fruit, potatoes, baked goods, sweets, juice, oatmeal and beer.

You need to eliminate apples, oranges, grapes, bananas, peaches, watermelon, pineapple, lemons, pears, melon, cherries, limes, plums, grapefruits, mango, and many more.

Most grains including rice, rye, oats, quinoa, corn, bulgur, amaranth, barley, wheat, millet, sprouted grains and buckwheat.

Starches including all types of bread, pasta, corn, rice, bagels, cereals, crackers, pizza, muesli, oatmeal, flour, popcorn and granola.

Beans including black, kidney, pinto, navy, soybeans as well as lentils, chickpeas and peas.

Real sugars and sweeteners such as cane sugar, agave nectar, maple syrup, agave nectar, honey, aspartame, Splenda, aspartame, corn syrup and saccharin.

Sweets including chocolate, candies, cakes, tarts, pies, buns, pastries, ice cream, puddings, custard and cookies.

You need to avoid the following cooking oils including canola, sesame, sunflower, grapeseed, soybean and peanut oil.

When it comes to alcohol you need to exclude sweet wine and alcoholic drinks, beer and cider.

Ketchup, tomato sauce, BBQ sauce, some salad dressings and hot sauces that contain added sugar all should be eliminated on the keto diet.

Finally, there is the low-fat dairy products such as mozzarella cheese, fat-free yoghurts, low-fat cheeses, cream cheese and skimmed milk should all be swapped for the high-fat versions.

Before you embark on the keto diet or any extreme weight loss play you should consult your doctor. Although the keto diet can include some foods i.e. broccoli you do have to say goodbye to many others.

PREPARING FOR YOUR KETO DIET

Like many diets you can improve the chance of success with some simple planning. The tips below are sure to help you on your way to a new and healthier you!

Prepare Your Kitchen

Before you begin a ketogenic diet, you need to get rid of any temptation that you may have in your cupboards. High carbohydrate products are too easy to grab eat without thinking and when your resolve is weak, and you will only stop craving carbs when your body reaches ketosis.

Stock up

You need to replace the high carbohydrate foods that you throw out, and you should start by stocking ketogenic staples such as oil, meats with plenty of fat, butter and make sure your cupboards are stocked with all the cooking ingredients you will need to create new low carbohydrate meals.

Be sure to stock up on electrolytes, natural sweetener and multivitamins as these will be your insurance to help prevent failure. You should ideally be getting your nutrients/electrolytes from your food, but no one is perfect, and therefore you need to keep these things at hand to help you through any rough patches.

Education

Learn everything you can about Ketogenic diets, there are some informative books that have been written by scientists and doctors which you should use for reference and ideas.

Never Shop when you are Hungry

Prior to shopping be sure you have eaten a small meal with plenty of fat as this will stop you from caving in and giving into cravings just because you are hungry. If you find it difficult shop online and plan your meals so that you only order things you want.

Keep drinking

When you begin a keto diet you much make sure to drink plenty of water as it is not only hydrated but it will help your body to get rid of toxins that have built up over time. It may not sound right but water refrains you from retaining water.

Work Out Your Correct Food Information

It is important that you know the exact ratios of protein, fat and carbohydrate that you can consume and how they fit into your diet plan.

The most important thing is to believe in yourself and before you know it, your keto diet will be second nature. The benefits of a slow cooker when following a keto diet

BREAKFAST

BREAKFAST CASSEROLE

Time: 1 ¾ hours / Serving 4

Net Carbs: 5% (6.1g / 0.22oz) Fiber: 0.9% (2.1g/0.007oz) Fat: 64.1% (9.8g/0.54oz)

Protein: 30% (22.9g/0.82oz) Kcal:313

INGREDIENTS:

- ◆ 6 large eggs
- ◆ 90g / 3.2 oz bacon slices
- ◆ 30g / 1.1oz chopped shallots
- ◆ 75 g/ 2.7 oz chopped red bell pepper
- ◆ 70 g/ 2.5 oz chopped white mushrooms
- ◆ 160 g/ 5.6 oz of kale, shredded finely
- ◆ 15 g/ 0.5 oz butter or ghee
- ◆ 90 g/ 3.2 oz Parmesan cheese shredded - or substitute for a cheese of choice
- ◆ Salt and pepper - to season

INSTRUCTIONS:

1. Remove the stems from the kale and chop in small pieces

2. Cook bacon until crispy, add the red pepper, mushroom and shallot, sauté until soft

3. Add the kale and turn off the heat, so kale wilts

4. Beat eggs, and add the salt and pepper

5. Select the high heat on your slow cooker and put the butter inside to melt, once melted brush the inside of the slow cooker

6. Add the sautéed vegetables to the slow cooker

7. Sprinkle the cheese over the vegetables then add the egg mix

8. Thoroughly stir the ingredients and cook at high setting for 2 hours or on low for 6 hours

BREKKIE BAKE

Time: 2 hours & 15 mins / Serving 12

Net Carbs: 0% (2g / 0.07oz) Fat: 33% (60g /2.17oz)

Protein: 64% (38g / 1.34oz) Kcal: 518

INGREDIENTS:

- ♦ 2 lbs / 32oz ground sausage
- ♦ 600g / 4 cups cheese
- ♦ 12 large eggs
- ♦ 75g / ½ cup sweet red pepper chopped
- ♦ 75g / ½ cup onion chopped
- ♦ 1 tsp salt
- ♦ 75g / ½ cup heavy cream
- ♦ ½ tsp freshly ground black pepper
- ♦ 1 packet of bacon

INSTRUCTIONS:

1. Cook the bacon in a skillet until crisp, leave to cool and then crumble

2. Use the skillet and cook the red peppers and onions for 3 minutes, add sausage and brown to crumble

3. Combine the cream, eggs, salt, and pepper and which until smooth

4. Add the sausage mix to the bottom of the slow cooker

5. Add 300g/2 cups of cheese on the top of the sausage, add the bacon and then top with the egg mix, and top with the final 300g/2 cups of cheese

6. Cook at a high heat for two hours then serve

BAKED BREAKFAST

Time: 2 hours 15 minutes / Serving 12

Net Carbs: 2g / 0.07oz Fat: 40g / 1.41oz

Protein: 34g / 1.20oz Kcal: 518

INGREDIENTS:

- ◆ 2lbs / 32oz ground sausage meat
- ◆ 4 cups/48oz of cheddar cheese
- ◆ 12 large eggs
- ◆ ½ cup / 6oz sweet red peppers chopped
- ◆ ½ cup / 6oz onion chopped
- ◆ 1 tsp / 5ml salt
- ◆ ½ cup / 6oz cream
- ◆ ½ tsp / 2.5 ml black pepper freshly ground
- ◆ 1 packet bacon

INSTRUCTIONS:

1. Cook bacon in skillet until crisp, cool, crumble and out to the side

2. Using the skillet with grease from the bacon to cook the onion and red peppers for 3 minutes

3. Add the sausage and brown until the mix is crumbled

4. Combine the eggs, cream, salt and pepper and whisk until smooth

5. Place the sausage mix into the bottom of your slow cooker

6. Top with 2 cups/24oz of cheese

7. Add the bacon to create a layer

8. Top with the egg mix

9. Create the final layer with the last 2 cups/24oz of cheese

10. Cook in the slow cooker for 2 hours, serve and enjoy

BREAKFAST ENCHILADAS

Time: 25 minutes / Serving 4

Net Carbs: 6.08g / 0.21oz Fat: 42.55g / 1.50oz

Protein: 27.3g / 0.96oz Kcal: 525

INGREDIENTS:

- 6 large eggs
- 60ml / ¼ cup heavy whipping cream
- ½ tsp / 2.5 ml salt
- ½ tsp / 2.5 ml garlic powder
- ½ tsp / 2.5 ml chili powder
- ¼ tsp / 1.25 ml black pepper
- ½ lb/ 8 oz ground sausage
- 180ml / ¾ cup enchilada sauce
- 375ml / 1½ cups shredded cheddar cheese

INSTRUCTIONS:

1. Turn your oven on to 400F and preheat a small skillet

2. Add the eggs, cream, salt, chili, and garlic powder together with black pepper and whisk

3. Pour 60ml / ¼ cup portions of the mixture into the pan and cover, cooked for 4 minutes, and then repeat with the other batter to create the rest of the chips

4. Add the cheese and sausage to your tortilla roll and place them in the slow cooker

5. Pour the enchilada sauce onto the mix making sure you cover all the egg

6. Top with the rest of the cheese and bake for 15 minutes

MEXICAN CASSEROLE BREAKFAST

Time: 5 hours 15 minutes / Serving 10
Net Carbs: 20g / 0.70oz Fat: 38g / 1.34oz
Protein: 29g / 1.02oz Kcal: 540

INGREDIENTS:

- 1 cup / 12oz ground pork
- ½ tsp / 1.25ml powdered garlic
- ½ tsp / 1.25ml coriander
- 1 tsp / 5ml powdered chili
- 1 tsp / 5ml cumin
- ¼ tsp / 0.65ml salt
- ¼ tsp / 0.65ml pepper
- 1 cup / 12oz Salsa
- 10 medium eggs
- 1 cup / 12oz cream
- 1 cup / 12oz Mexican Blend cheese

INSTRUCTIONS:

1. Cook the pork until browned

2. Add the salsa and seasoning and leave to cool

3. Whisk the cream and eggs

4. Combine the pork, egg mix and cream

5. Grease the bottom of the slow cooker and pour in the mixture

6. Cook on high for 2 ½ hours or on low for 5 hours

HAM & CHEESE WAFFLE

Time: 3 hours / Serving 2
Net Carbs: 37g / 1.3oz Fat: 42g / 1.48oz
Protein: 38g / 1.34oz Kcal: 683

INGREDIENTS:

- 1 cup / 12oz cubed ham
- 6 eggs
- 2 cups / 500ml milk
- ½ tsp / 1.25ml paprika
- 1 tsp / 5ml salt
- 226g / 8oz Extra mature cheddar grated
- 300g / 10.5oz waffles cut in cubes
- Maple Syrup if desired for serving

INSTRUCTIONS:

1. Mix the eggs, milk, paprika and salt

2. In a slow cooker layer ½ of the waffle mix, then ½ ham and ½ grated cheese

3. Repeat as point 2

4. Pour the egg mix over

5. Cook on high for 3 hours

LUNCH

APRICOT, CHICKEN AND RICE POT

Time: 2 hours 45 minutes / Serving 2

Net Carbs: 70g / 2.46oz Fat: 38.8g /1.37oz

Protein: 29g / 1.02oz Kcal: 473

INGREDIENTS:

- 1 cup / 225g of rice
- 4 chicken thighs, boneless and skinned
- 1 cup / 150g chopped onion
- 2 ½ cups / 600ml chicken broth
- 1 tsp / 4.2g paprika
- 1 tsp / 4.2g oregano
- 1 cup / 140g of mixed frozen peas and carrots
- ¼ tsp / 0.65ml salt
- ¼ tsp / 0.65ml pepper
- ½ tsp / 1.2ml garlic minced
- 1 cup / 225g pineapple
- 1 tablespoon / 17.5ml Olive oil
- 15 apricots dried and chopped

INSTRUCTIONS:

1. Add the oil to your slow cooker

2. Sauté the onions for 3 minutes until soft then stir in the garlic

3. Add the onions and garlic with the chicken broth, paprika, salt and pepper to the slow cooker

4. Stir in the rice and top with the chicken thighs

SLOW COOKED CHICKEN BREAST

Time: 1 hour 25 minutes / Serving 3
Net Carbs: 2g / 0.07oz Fat: 13g / 0.46oz
Protein: 35g / 1.23oz Kcal: 282

INGREDIENTS:

- 1lb / 16oz chicken fillets boneless and skinless
- 180ml / 6oz chicken stock
- 2 tbsp olive oil
- 1 tsp mixed dried herbs
- ½ tsp ground coriander
- ½ tsp ground ginger
- ½ tsp ground garlic
- Salt and Pepper to taste

INSTRUCTIONS:

1. Mix herbs, ginger, coriander, paprika, garlic, salt, pepper, 1 tablespoon of oil and 2 tablespoons of chicken stock to create a paste

2. Coat the chicken fillets with the paste and fry until they are brown on either side

3. Place the chicken into the slow cooker and add the remaining stock

4. Cook on a low heat for 1 hour and 15 minutes

5. Plate up and enjoy

INSTANT MEATBALLS

Time: 45 minutes / Serving 8
Net Carbs: 6g / 0.21oz Fat: 25g / 0.08oz
Protein: 20g / 0.70oz Kcal: 333

INGREDIENTS:

- 1 ½ lb / 24oz ground turkey or beef
- 2 tablespoons water
- 2 tablespoons parsley chopped
- 2 finely chopped spring onions
- ½ cup / 8oz almond flour
- 1 teaspoon dried oregano
- 1 teaspoon pureed garlic
- 2 eggs
- Salt to taste
- Sauce
- 2 x 14oz tins of diced tomatoes
- 1 tablespoon of olive oil
- 1 tablespoon red wine vinegar
- 3 tablespoons of water
- 1 teaspoon Italian seasoning

INSTRUCTIONS:

1. Combine all the meatball ingredients together until well mixed
2. Form the balls
3. Add the oil to your slow cooker then add the meatballs taking care not to squash them
4. Pour the water, vinegar, tomatoes, and herbs over the balls
5. Cook on high heat for 45 minutes

INSTANT STEAK FAJITAS

Time: 3 hours & 10 minutes / Serving 6
Net Carbs: 7.7g / 0.27oz Fat: 8.1g / 0.28oz
Protein: 33.8g / 1.19oz Kcal: 242

INGREDIENTS:

- ◆ 2lbs / 32oz sliced beef
- ◆ 425g / 15oz diced tomatoes
- ◆ ¼ cup / 2oz beef broth
- ◆ 2 sliced bell peppers
- ◆ 1 sliced onion
- ◆ 2 tablespoons fajita seasoning
- ◆ 1 tablespoon of oil

INSTRUCTIONS:

1. Add all ingredients to your slow cooker and mix well

2. Cook on high for 3 hours / on low for 6 hours

3. Enjoy!

OODLES ZOODLES & MEATBALLS

Time: 4 hours & 10 minutes / Serving 4

Net Carbs: 9g / 0.32oz Fat: 5.8g / 0.20oz

Protein: 29.7g / 1.05oz Kcal: 218

INGREDIENTS:

The Zoodles

♦ 3 Zucchini to create the Oodles of Zoodles

♦ 2 teaspoons of oil

The Sauce

♦ 28 oz/ 795g of crushed tomatoes

♦ 1 minced garlic clove

♦ Salt & Pepper to taste

The Meatballs

♦ 1lb / 16oz ground meat

♦ 1 egg

♦ 2 tablespoons seasoning (Italian)

♦ ½ teaspoon of salt

♦ ¼ teaspoon of pepper

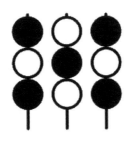

INSTRUCTIONS:

1. Add all the ingredients for the sauce to the slow cooker and mix thoroughly

2. Add the meatball ingredients to a bowl and mix well

3. Form the mixture into 10 – 12 meatballs

4. Add the meatballs to the slow cooker

5. Using a peeler create zoodles from the Zucchi (or purchase these ready done)

6. Cook on high for 2 – 3 hours or on low for 4 – 6 hours

7. Add the zoodles to the slow cooker for the last 10 minutes until these are tender

PULLED PORK FROM MEXICO

Time: 8 hours 40 minutes / Serving 11

Net Carbs: 1g / 0.03oz Fat: 7g / 0.25oz

Protein: 20g / 0.70oz Kcal: 160

INGREDIENTS:

- ◆ 2 ½ lbs / 40oz pork shoulder boneless and trimmed
- ◆ ¾ cup / 200ml chicken broth reduced sodium
- ◆ 6 garlic cloves cut to slithers
- ◆ 1 ½ teaspoons of cumin
- ◆ ½ teaspoon of sazon
- ◆ Black pepper to taste
- ◆ ¼ teaspoon of dry oregano
- ◆ 2 – 3 chipotle peppers
- ◆ 2 teaspoons of kosher salt
- ◆ 2 bay leaves
- ◆ ¼ teaspoon dry adobo seasoning

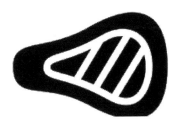

INSTRUCTION:

1. Season the pork using the salt and pepper

2. Brown the pork all over for about 8 minutes

3. Insert a blade into the pork and make small holes to insert the garlic completely into the meat

4. Season the pork with the oregano, cumin, adobo, and sazon

5. Add the chicken broth to the slow cooker with the bay leaves and peppers

6. Place the pork into the slow cooker cover, and cook on low for 8 hours

7. After the 8 hours use two forks to shred the pork and mix this well with the juices at the bottom of the pot

8. Remove the bay leaves and add more salt and cumin if desired

9. Cook for a further 30 minutes

10. Serve and enjoy

CHILI TIME

Time: 8 hours 15 minutes / Serving 10

Net Carbs: 13g / 0.46oz Fat:18g / 0.81oz

Protein: 23g / 0.70oz Kcal: 306

INGREDIENTS:

- 2 ½ lbs / 40 oz ground beef
- 2 x 15oz / 2 x 440ml cans of tomatoes diced
- 6oz / 175ml tomato paste
- 4 oz / 110ml green chiles
- 1 small, chopped onion
- 8 cloves of minced garlic
- 2 tablespoons of Worcester sauce
- ½ cup / 170g powdered chili
- 2 tablespoons of cumin
- 1 tablespoon of oregano dried
- 1 teaspoon of black pepper
- 1 teaspoon of sea salt

INSTRUCTIONS:

1. Over a high heat cook the onion for about 5 minutes then add the garlic and cook for a further 1 minute

2. Add the beef and cooked for 10 minutes until browned

3. Transfer the beef to the slow cooker and add the rest of the ingredients and stir until thoroughly combined

4. Cook for 8 hours on low or 4 hours on high

5. Serve and enjoy

STUFFED CABBAGE ROLLS

Time: 10 hours / Serving 4
Net Carbs: 37g / 1.30oz Fat:26g / 0.92oz
Protein: 28g / 0.99oz Kcal: 484

INGREDIENTS:

- 1lb / 16oz of ground beef
- 1/3 cup / 113g uncooked reg. rice
- 1 egg
- ¼ teaspoon of pepper
- 2 teaspoons of sugar
- 1 tin 15oz / 425g diced tomatoes
- Head of cabbage
- 1 onion grated
- 1 teaspoon of salt
- ¼ teaspoon of hot flaked peppers
- 1 tin 8oz / 225g tomato sauce

INSTRUCTIONS:

1. Pull 12 leaves from the cabbage head and place in boiling water

2. Cook the cabbage until it is limp then drain and set aside

3. Mix the ground beef, rice, egg, onion, salt, and pepper

4. Lay one cabbage leaf out and place some mixture in it then fold in the sides to create a cabbage roll, add to the slow cooker, and repeat until all the cabbage is used

5. Mix the pepper flakes, sugar, diced tomatoes, and tomato sauce until fully combined

6. Pour over the cabbage rolls and cook on low for 10 hours

BAKED LOADED POTATO SOUP

Time: 10 hours / Serving 6

Net Carbs: 39g / 1.37oz Fat: 37g / 1.30oz

Protein: 17g / 0.60oz Kcal: 553

INGREDIENTS:

- 6 baking potatoes
- 4 cups / 1000ml chicken broth
- ¼ cup / 85g of butter
- 1 teaspoon of black pepper
- 1 cup / 340g shredded cheese
- 1 cup / 250ml of sour cream
- Cheddar cheese, for sprinkling if desired
- 1 onion
- 3 cloves of garlic
- 2 ½ teaspoon of salt
- 1 cup / 250ml cream
- 3 tablespoons fresh chopped chives
- 8 fried and crumbled bacon slices

INSTRUCTIONS:

1. Peel the potatoes and cut them into ½ "cubes

2. Chop the onions and press or crush the garlic

3. Add the potatoes broth, garlic, onion, butter, salt, and pepper to the slow cooker

4. Cook on low for 4 hours so the potatoes are tender

5. Mash the ingredients until it is chunky and not totally smashed

6. Stir in the cream, cheese and chives and turn the slow cooker to high for a further 15 minutes

7. Serve with a dollop of sour cream, crumbled bacon, shredded cheese if desired

DINNER

BROCCOLI, SAUSAGE, CHEESY SOUP

Time: 2 - 3 hours / Serving 4

Net Carbs: 7g / 0.25oz Fat: 7g / 0.25oz

Protein: 15g / 0.53oz Kcal 229

INGREDIENTS:

- ♦ ½ lb / 8oz breakfast sausage
- ♦ 2 cups / 680g broccoli florets
- ♦ 1 cup / 340g carrots diced
- ♦ ½ lb / 8oz cubed velveeta
- ♦ 2 cups / 500ml beef stock
- ♦ 2 tablespoons of powdered garlic
- ♦ 1 cup / 340g shredded cheese

INSTRUCTIONS:

1. Brown the sausage, add to slow cooker with all if the ingredients except the cheese

2. Cook on a low heat for 2 – 3 hours

3. Add the cheese to the now soup mix and serve

SLOW SALMON

Time: 2 hours / Serving 6
Net Carbs: 6.29g / 0.22oz Fat: 15.3g / 0.54oz
Protein: 23.3g / 0.82oz Kcal:261

INGREDIENTS:

- ◆ 1 – 2lbs / 16 – 32oz salmon fillets with skin on
- ◆ 1 – 1 ½ cups / 225g – 337g of chosen liquid (broth, cider, water etc.)
- ◆ Salt
- ◆ Fresh black pepper
- ◆ Spices (if desired)
- ◆ Sliced lemon (if desired)
- ◆ Sliced aromatic vegetables, onions, celery etc. (if desired)

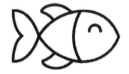

INSTRUCTIONS:

1. Begin by cutting the salmon into number of fillets

2. Sprinkle the fillets with fresh salt and pepper and season the flesh side

3. Sprinkle any other spices if you are using them, use your fingers to rub everything in

4. Line your slow cooker using a square of foil or parchment and place in the slow cooker

5. Put your vegetables and spices in the bottom if you are using them

6. Place a layer of lemon slices if required this will add flavour

7. Place your first layer of salmon putting the larger skin side down

8. Add another layer complete with additional lemon and vegetables

9. Add the liquid you have chosen to your slow cooker

10. Cook on low setting for 1 – 2 hours

11. Remove from the slow cooker and remove liquid

12. Serve immediately or cool and refrigerate

PORK TENDERLOIN

Time: 4 hours / Serving 8

Net Carbs: 0g / 0oz Fat: 7g / 0.25oz

Protein: 23g / 0.81oz Kcal: 169

INGREDIENTS:

- ♦ 2 - 3 lb / 32oz – 48oz pork tenderloin
- ♦ 4 garlic cloves chopped
- ♦ Juice of one lemon
- ♦ 2 tbsp / 30ml olive oil
- ♦ 1 tsp / 5ml salt
- ♦ 1 tsp / 5ml pepper
- ♦ ½ - 1 tsp / 2.5ml – 5ml gravy thickening

INSTRUCTIONS:

1. Place the pork in slow cooker

2. Add the garlic, olive oil, salt, pepper and lemon juice to the pork and mix

3. Cover and cook for 3 – 4 hours

4. Remove the pork from the slow cooker and sprinkle gravy thickener then whisk

5. Once the gravy has thickened, cut the pork, and serve with gravy

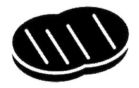

BEEF SHORT RIBS

Time: 6 hours & 30 mins / Serving 12
Net Carbs: 2g / 0.07oz Fat: 42g / 1.48oz
Protein: 16g / 0.56oz Kcal: 489

INGREDIENTS:

- 4 lbs / 64oz boneless beef short ribs cut into 2" pieces
- 2 tbsp / 30ml olive oil
- 250ml / 1 cup beef broth
- 375ml / 1 ½ cup onion chopped
- 3 cloves of minced garlic
- 2 tbsp / 30ml Worcestershire sauce
- 2 tbsp / 30ml tomato paste
- 375ml / 1 ½ cup red wine
- Salt & Pepper

INSTRUCTIONS:

1. Heat the oil and generously season the ribs with salt and pepper
2. Put half of the ribs onto the skillet to brown, season and then turn to brown the other side
3. Set these to one side with the other meat
4. Add your broth to your slow cooker and add the ribs
5. Add the remaining ingredients to the skillet and boil
6. Cook until the onion is soft and then pour this over the ribs
7. Cook on a high for 4 – 6 hours

CHILI STEAK

Time: 6 hours / Serving 12
Net Carbs: 4.79g / 0.17oz Fat: 37.26g / 1.31oz
Protein: 16g / 0.56oz Kcal: 478

INGREDIENTS:

- ♦ 2 ½ lbs / 40 oz steak, in 1" cubes
- ♦ 1 tbsp / 15ml of ancho chili powder
- ♦ ½ tsp / 2.5ml ground cumin
- ♦ ½ tsp / 2.5ml salt
- ♦ ¼ tsp / 1.25 ml of ground cayenne pepper
- ♦ ¼ tsp / 1.25 ml of ground black pepper
- ♦ ½ cup / 170g sliced leeks
- ♦ 500ml / 2 cups canned tomatoes, include the juice
- ♦ 250ml / 1 cup of chicken or beef stock

INSTRUCTIONS:

1. Place all the ingredients into your slow cooker

2. Stir until well mixed and cook on high for approximately 6 hours or until the steak is soft

3. With a fork break any of the tomatoes that are still whole and shred the steak if needed

4. Serve and enjoy

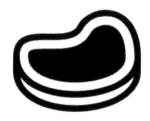

PERFECT PULLED PORK

Time: 8 hours / Serving 10

Net Carbs: 6.5g / 0.23oz Fat: 1.5g / 0.05oz

Protein: 11g / 0.39oz Kcal: 93

INGREDIENTS:

- 1lb / 16oz tenderloin pork
- 1 can / 28oz crushed tomatoes
- 1 small jar / 7oz drained red roasted peppers
- 5 cloves of smashed garlic
- 1 teaspoon of olive oil
- 1 tsp kosher salt
- 2 sprigs of thyme & 2 bay leaves
- 1 tablespoon chopped parsley
- Black pepper to season

INSTRUCTIONS:

1. Season pork using the salt and pepper

2. Sauté the garlic in the oil until brown then remove

3. Add the pork and brown for 2 minutes each side

4. Put the pork into the slow cooker with the garlic and all the other ingredients, keep back half of the chopped parsley

5. Cook on a low heat for 8 hours

6. Remove bay leaves, shred the pork, and sprinkle the remaining parsley over the dish

MASALA CHICKEN

Time: 4 hours / Serving 4

Net Carbs: 7g / 0.25oz Fat: 5g / 0.18oz

Protein: 33g / 1.16oz Kcal: 312

INGREDIENTS:

- 4 medium chicken breasts
- 225g / 8oz sliced button mushrooms
- 1 cup / 235ml marsala dry wine
- ½ cup / 118ml heavy whipping cream
- Salt & Pepper to season
- Dash of oil

INSTRUCTIONS:

1. Add small amount of oil to your slow cooker

2. Add the chicken to the bottom of the slow cooker

3. Layer the seasonings and mushrooms on top of the chicken and cover with the wine

4. Cook for 3 hours and 30 minutes on high

5. Remove the chicken and mushrooms from the slow cooker

6. Stir in the cream and whisk until the cream thickens

7. Put the chicken and mushrooms back into the slow cooker and cook for a further ½ hour

8. Serve and enjoy

PICADILLO POT

Time: 3 hours & 30 minutes / Serving 11
Net Carbs: 5g / 0.18oz Fat: 8.5g / 0.30oz
Protein: 28g / 0.99oz Kcal: 207

INGREDIENTS:

- ♦ 2 ½ lbs / 40oz lean ground beef
- ♦ 1 cup / 340g onion minced
- ♦ 1 cup / 340g red bell peppers minced
- ♦ 1 diced tomato
- ♦ 8oz / 225g tin of tomato sauce
- ♦ Salt & pepper to taste
- ♦ ¼ cup / 85g cilantro minced
- ♦ ¼ cup / 85g green olives
- ♦ 1 ½ teaspoons cumin ground
- ♦ ¼ teaspoon powdered garlic
- ♦ 2 bay leaves

INSTRUCTIONS:

1. Brown the meat and season with salt and pepper

2. Use wooden spoon to break the meat up into small chunks

3. Drain the excess liquid from the pan used to cook the meat and add the garlic, bell peppers and onions to the meat and cook for a further 3 ½ minutes

4. Place the meat into your slow cooker and add the rest of the Ingredients

5. Cook on High for 3 ½ hours

PORK & RICE CHOPS

Time: 8 hours / Serving 4

Net Carbs: 48g / 1.69oz Fat: 21g / 0.74oz

Protein: 29g / 1.02oz Kcal: 508

INGREDIENTS:

- ♦ 4 pork chops or steaks
- ♦ 1 packet of onion soup powder
- ♦ 2 cups / 500ml of water
- ♦ 1 cup /340g of uncooked rice
- ♦ 1 can / 300g cream of mushroom soup

INSTRUCTIONS:

1. Brown the pork

2. Add the rice to the slow cooker

3. Sprinkle 1/3 of the onion soup over it and pour the water over the top

4. Cook on low for 8 hours

DESSERTS

DESSERTS

LUSCIOUS LEMON CAKE

Time: 3 hours / Serving 8
Net Carbs: 10g / 0.35oz Fat: 32g / 1.13oz
Protein: 7g / 0.25oz Kcal: 347

INGREDIENTS:

For the Cake

- ◆ 1 ½ cups / 510 g of Almond flour
- ◆ 1 ½ cups / 510 g of Coconut flour
- ◆ 2 teaspoons of Baking Powder
- ◆ 6 tablespoons of Swerve
- ◆ ½ cup / 170g of melted butter
- ◆ ½ cup / 125ml of cream (whipping)
- ◆ 2 lemons for the zest and the juice
- ◆ 2 eggs

Cake Topping

- ◆ 3 tablespoons of Swerve
- ◆ ½ cup / 125ml boiled water
- ◆ 2 tablespoons / g melted butter
- ◆ 2 tablespoons / ml lemon juice

INSTRUCTIONS:

For the Cake

1. In a bowl mix the almond and coconut flour, swerve, and baking powder

2. Whisk the butter, cream, zest and juice from the lemon and an egg

3. Add the two mixes (step 1 & 2) together and combine thoroughly

4. Line your slow cooker with foil and spread the cake mixture onto it

Cake Topping

1. Combine all ingredients and pour over the top of the cake mix in the slow cooker

2. Cook in the slow cooker for 2 – 3 hours (insert a toothpick into the center of the cake and if this comes out clean the cake is ready)

3. Serve with fresh fruit and whipped cream

TASTY DARK CHOCOLATE CAKE

Time: 2 ½ hours / Serving 10
Net Carbs: 8.4g / 0.30oz Fat: 17g / 0.60oz
Protein: 7.4g / 0.26oz Kcal: 205

INGREDIENTS:

- ◆ 1 cup / 340g of almond flour + an additional 2 tablespoons of almond flour
- ◆ ½ cup / 170g Swerve Granular Sweetener
- ◆ ½ cup / 170g of cocoa powder
- ◆ 3 tablespoons of egg white powdered protein
- ◆ 1 ½ teaspoons of baking powder
- ◆ ¼ teaspoon of salt
- ◆ 6 tablespoons of melted butter
- ◆ 3 eggs
- ◆ 2/3 cups / 6ml of almond milk unsweetened
- ◆ ¾ teaspoon of vanilla extract
- ◆ 1/3 cup / 113g of chocolate chips (sugar free)

INSTRUCTIONS:

1. Grease the inside of your slow cooker well

2. Whisk the almond flour, sweetener, protein powder, cocoa powder, salt, and baking powder

3. Stir in the eggs, butter, almond milk, vanilla extract, and chocolate chips

4. Pour into your slow cooker and cook on a low heat for 2 ½ hours (if you want a gooier consistency it will be ready in 2 hours)

5. Turn off your slow cooker and leave the cake to cool for 30 minutes

6. Serve and enjoy

CHOCOLATE & RASPBERRY CAKE

Time: 3 ½ hours / Serving 10

Carbs: 6.8 g / 0.24oz Fat: 26.6g / 0.94oz

Protein: 4.5g / 0.16oz Kcal: 242

INGREDIENTS:

- 1 cup / 340g Hazelnut flour
- ½ cup / 170g of sweetener
- ¼ cup / 85g of cocoa powder unsweetened
- 1 ½ teaspoons of baking powder
- ¼ teaspoon of salt
- 1 tablespoon of expresso coffee powder
- 2 oz / 56g of chopped unsweetened chocolate
- ½ cup / 170g of unsalted butter cut in chunks
- 3 large eggs
- ½ cup / 125ml unsweetened almond milk
- 2 teaspoons of vanilla extract
- 1 cup / 340g of Raspberries

INSTRUCTIONS:

1. Oil the inside of your slow cooker

2. Mix the flour, sweetener, cocoa powder, salt, expresso powder and baking powder and set to one side

3. Melt the unsweetened chocolate and butter until combined and let cool

4. Beat the eggs until they are frothy, beat the cream in slowly, add the extract then pour all the wet ingredients in with the dry and mix thoroughly

5. Once the chocolate has cooled (you want to be sure it will not cook the eggs) pour into the batter and combine

6. Fold the raspberries into the batter

7. Pour the batter into the slow cooker and spread so it is even

8. Place a piece of paper towel over the top of the slow cooker to ensure no condensation falls onto the cake during cooking or when you remove the lid

9. Cook on low for 3 ½ hours, then cool and serve

SKINNY MINT CHOCOLATE CAKE

Time: 3 hours & 45 minutes / Serving 8

Net Carbs: 8g / 0.28oz Fat: 19g / 0.67oz

Protein: 6g / 0.21oz Kcal: 214

INGREDIENTS:

- 1 cup / 125g almond flour
- ½ cup / 62.5g sweetener
- ¼ cup / 31.25g cocoa powder sugar free
- 1½ teaspoons of baking powder
- ¼ teaspoon of salt
- 3 eggs
- 6 tablespoons of melted butter (no salt)
- 2/3 cup / 62ml of almond milk unsweetened
- ½ teaspoon of peppermint extract
- ¼ teaspoon of cinnamon
- 1/3 mini chocolate chips (low carb)

INSTRUCTIONS:

1. Combine the flour, sweetener, cocoa powder, baking powder and salt

2. Beat the eggs and add them to the melted butter, almond milk, peppermint extract and chocolate chips

3. Grease the bowl of your slow cooker then pour the batter into the pot and cook on a low setting for 3 hours 15 minutes

4. Let the cake cool for 30 minutes and serve warm

FINGERS OF FUDGE

Time: 1 hour 30 minutes / Serving 25

Net Carbs: 0g / 0oz Fat: 9g / 0.32oz

Protein: 0g / 0oz Kcal: 98

INGREDIENTS:

- 1 cup / 250ml coconut milk full fat
- 2 ½ cups / 810g chocolate chips sugar free
- 1 teaspoon vanilla extract
- 2 teaspoons of stevia liquid to taste
- 1/8 teaspoon of salt

INSTRUCTIONS:

1. Line 8x8" baking dish with parchment paper

2. Add the coconut milk to your slow cooker and add the vanilla, chocolate chips, stevia and salt and combine thoroughly

3. Cover the slow cooker with a paper towel and put on the lid slightly ajar so that the steam can escape as water and chocolate do not mix well

4. Cook for 1 ½ hours on low then turn off and stir the mixture so that it is smooth

5. Spread the fudge mixture onto the prepared baking dish

6. Chill for 1 hour in the fridge or until it is firm

LEMON AND BURSTING LEMON CUSTARD CAKE

Time: 3 hours 15 minutes / Serving 12
Net Carbs: 4g / 0.14oz Fat: 17g / 0.60oz
Protein: 4g / 0.14oz Kcal: 191

INGREDIENTS:

♦ ½ cup / 170g of coconut flour

♦ 6 eggs separated

♦ 1/3 cup / 80ml lemon juice

♦ 2 teaspoons of lemon zest

♦ 1 teaspoon of liquid stevia

♦ ½ teaspoon of salt

♦ 2 cups / 500ml of heavy cream

♦ ½ cup / 170g of blueberries (fresh)

INSTRUCTIONS:

1. Add the egg whites in a mixer and mix until they form stiff peaks, put to one side

2. Whisk the yolks and all remaining ingredients except the blueberries

3. Fold the egg whites into the batter until thoroughly combined

4. Grease your slow cooker and pour the mixture into the pot

5. Sprinkle the blueberries on top of the batter mix

6. Cover and cook on a low heat for 3 hours

7. Remove the cover of the slow cooker and cool for 1 hour, chill then enjoy

PUMPKIN BARS

Time: 3 Hours 15 minutes / Serving 16 bars
Net Carbs: 6g / 0.21oz Fat: 15g / 0.53oz
Protein: 4g / 0.14oz Kcal: 169

INGREDIENTS:

For the Crust

♦ ¾ cup / 255g shredded coconut

♦ ¼ cup / 85g cocoa powder unsweetened

♦ ½ cup / 170g sunflower seed flour

♦ ¼ teaspoon of salt

♦ ¼ cup / 85g of sweetener

♦ 4 tablespoons softened unsalted butter

For the Filling

♦ 1 can / 125ml of pumpkin puree

♦ 1 can / 125ml of cream

♦ 6 eggs

♦ ½ teaspoon of salt

♦ 1 tablespoon pumpkin pie spice

♦ 1 tablespoon vanilla extract

♦ 2 tablespoons of cinnamon stevia liquid

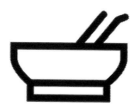

INSTRUCTIONS:

For the Crust

1. Add all the crust ingredients into a processor to create fine crumbs

2. Grease the bottom of your slow cooker

3. Press the crust mixture into the bottom of your slow cooker as evenly as you can

For the Filling

1. Put all the filling ingredients into a mixer and blend until thoroughly combined

2. Pour the mixture onto the crust in the slow cooker

3. Cover and cook on a low setting for 3 hours

4. Uncover and let the mixture cool and then place your slow cooker into the fridge for a further 3 hours

5. Slice and serve

COFFEE AND RASPBERRY CREAM CHEESECAKE

Time: 4 hours 15 minutes / Serving 12
Net Carbs: 6.95g / 0.25oz Fat: 19.18g / 0.68oz
Protein: 7.54g / 0.26oz Kcal: 239

INGREDIENTS:

Cake Batter

- 1 ¼ cups / 425g of almond flour
- ½ cup / 125ml of sweetener
- ¼ cup / 85g coconut flour
- ¼ cup / 85g vanilla protein powder
- 1 ½ teaspoons of baking powder
- ¼ teaspoon of salt
- 3 large eggs
- 6 tablespoons of melted butter
- 2/3 cup / 165ml of water
- ½ teaspoon of vanilla extract

Filling

- 8oz / 225g cream cheese
- 1/3 cup / 115g powdered sweetener
- 1 large egg
- 2 tablespoons of cream for whipping
- 1 ½ cup / 510g of fresh raspberries

INSTRUCTION:

1. Grease the inside of your slow cooker

2. To make the cake batter combine the almond and coconut flour, sweetener, powered protein, salt, and baking powder

3. Stir in the melted butter, eggs, and water until thoroughly combined then put to the side

4. Beat the cream cheese and sweetener for the filling until smooth, then beat in the egg, vanilla extract, and cream until well combined

5. Add about two thirds of the batter into the slow cooker then pour the cream cheese mixture over the batter and spread evenly

6. Sprinkle the cake mix with the raspberries then dot the remaining batter over the filling and some of the filling is still shown

7. Bake on the low setting for 4 hours

8. When the edges are golden brown, and the filling has just set turn off the slow cooker

9. Remove the inside of the cooker and allow the cake to cool fully before serving

RICH RICE PUDDING

Time: 4 hours 20 minutes / Serving 12

Net Carbs: 75g / 2.64oz Fat: 13g / 0.46oz

Protein: 16g / 0.56oz Kcal: 483

INGREDIENTS:

- 1 cup / 340g of uncooked white rice
- 8 cups / 2000ml of milk
- ½ cup / 125ml
- 1/4 teaspoon of salt
- 1 cup / 340g sugar
- 2 eggs
- 2 teaspoons of vanilla extract
- Cinnamon or Nutmeg

INSTRUCTIONS:

1. Combine the sugar, rice, and half of the milk into the slot cooker
2. Stir thoroughly, cover and cook on high for 4 hours
3. Mix the eggs, vanilla, salt, and remaining milk
4. Pour this into slow cooker and mix
5. Cover and cook for a further 20 minutes the pudding will thicken
6. Serve warm with nutmeg or cinnamon sprinkled over the top if desired

PEACH COBBLER & CRUNCHY OATY TOP

Time: 3 hours / Serving 8
Net Carbs: 38g / 1.34oz Fat: 18g / 0.63oz
Protein: 4g / 0.14oz Kcal: 324

INGREDIENTS:

- 2 lbs / 32 oz fresh sliced peaches
- 2/3 cup / 255g of all-purpose flour
- ½ teaspoon of ground cinnamon
- ¾ cup / 255g soft butter
- 2/3 cup / 255g of oats
- 2/3 cup / 255g light brown sugar
- ¼ teaspoon of ground nutmeg

INSTRUCTIONS:

1. Lay the peach slices at the bottom of the slow cooker
2. Combine the oats, sugar, flour, nutmeg. and cinnamon until thoroughly mixed
3. Add the butter and stir the mix until it equates to crumble
4. Top the peaches with the crumble
5. Cover the slow cooker
6. Cook on low for 3 hours
7. Serve and enjoy

14 DAY MEAL PLANNER

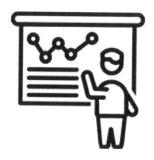

DAY ONE

Breakfast – Chocolate German Oatmeal

Time: 6 hours 5 minutes / Serving 6
Net Carbs: 39g / 1.37oz Fat: 19.18g / 0.68oz
Protein: 7.54g / 0.26oz Kcal: 267

INGREDIENTS:

- ◆ 2 cups / 680g Oats
- ◆ 13.5oz / 400ml can of coconut lite milk
- ◆ Brown sugar
- ◆ Chopped pecan nuts
- ◆ 7 cups / 1000ml of water
- ◆ ¼ cup unsweetened cocoa powder
- ◆ Shredded coconut sweetened

INSTRUCTIONS:

1. Grease the slow cooker

2. Mix the oats, water, coconut milk and cocoa powder

3. Pour into the slow cooker

4. Cook for 6 hours on a low setting

5. Top with pecan nuts, brown sugar and shredded coconut as preferred

Lunch - Slow Cooked Chicken Breast (See page 41)

Dinner – Slow Salmon (See page 55)

Dessert - Tasty Dark Chocolate Cake (See page 68)

DAY TWO

Breakfast – Breakfast Enchiladas (See page 36)

Lunch – Chili Time (See page 48)

Dinner – Perfect Pulled Pork (See page 60)

Dessert – Mocha Pudding

Time: 3 hours 30 minutes / Serving 6
Net Carbs: 3.76g / 0.13oz Fat: 39.81g / 1.40oz
Protein: 9.29g / 0.33oz Kcal: 413.5

INGREDIENTS:

- ♦ ¾ cup / 255g butter
- ♦ ½ cup / 125ml cream
- ♦ 1 teaspoon of vanilla extract
- ♦ 1/3 cup / 114g of almond flour
- ♦ 5 eggs
- ♦ 2oz / 55g unsweetened finely chopped chocolate
- ♦ 2 tablespoons of instant coffee granules
- ♦ 4 tablespoons of cocoa powder (unsweetened)
- ♦ 1/8 teaspoon of salt
- ♦ 2/3 Cup / 227g of sweetener granules

INSTRUCTIONS:

1. Grease the slow cooker with coconut oil spray

2. Melt the butter and unsweetened chocolate leave to cool

3. Whisk the cream, coffee granules and vanilla extract

4. Mix the cocoa powder with the almond flour and salt

5. Beat the eggs then add the granulated sweetener, beat for a further 5 minutes

6. Mix in the butter and chocolate (Step 2)

7. Stir the almond flour, cocoa, and salt into the mixture

8. Slowly add the cream, coffee, and vanilla

9. Transfer to the slow cooker

10. Place kitchen towel over the slow cooker and then add the lid (the paper towel is to ensure that the condensation does not drip into the pudding)

11. Cook for 3 hours on low

12. Serve with cream if desired

DAY THREE

Breakfast – Ham & Cheese Waffle (See page 38)

Lunch – Apricot, Chicken and Rice Pot (See page 40)

Dinner – Slow Cooker Greek Chicken

Time: 4 hours 15 minutes / Serving 6
Net Carbs: 4g / 0.14oz Fat: 36g / 1.27oz
Protein: 1g / 0.03oz Kcal: 452

INGREDIENTS:

♦ 2 lbs / 32 oz of chicken thighs (no skin or bones)

♦ 3 cloves of garlic

♦ ¼ teaspoon of lemon pepper

♦ 1 x 8oz / 235ml artichoke hearts marinated

♦ ½ sliced red onion

♦ ¼ cup / 90ml red wine vinegar

♦ 1 teaspoon oregano dried

♦ 1 tablespoon of arrowroot starch

♦ 2 tablespoons of olive oil

♦ ½ teaspoons of salt

♦ 1 x 12oz / 355 ml red peppers diced/drained

♦ 1 cup / 340g kalamata olives

♦ 2/3 cup / 180ml chicken broth

♦ Juice of ½ a lemon

♦ 1 teaspoon thyme dried

♦ 1 tablespoon chopped fresh basil

INSTRUCTIONS:

1. Mix half of the chicken broth with the lemon juice, vinegar, dried thyme, and oregano

2. Put the chicken and vegetable in the slow cooker and cover with the chicken broth (Step 1)

3. Cover the slow cooker and cook for 4 hours on low

4. Once cooked remove some of the liquid and add 1 tablespoon of the arrowroot starch to the juice, mix well and put it back into the slow cooker

5. Allow the sauce to thicken for about 15 minutes

6. Serve and enjoy

Dessert - Chocolate & Raspberry Cake (See page 70)

DAY FOUR

Breakfast - Brekkie Bake (See page 33)

Lunch – Taco Slow Soup

Time: 4 hours 20 minutes / Serving 10

Net Carbs: 4g / 0.14oz Fat: 36g / 1.27oz

Protein: 1g / 0.03oz Kcal: 452

INGREDIENTS:

♦ 2 lbs / 32 oz of ground beef

♦ 10 oz / 280g can of tomatoes diced

♦ 1 tablespoon of cumin

♦ ½ teaspoon of salt and pepper

♦ 3 cups / 750ml of beef broth

♦ ½ lb / 16 oz of cream cheese

♦ 1 tablespoon and 1 teaspoon chili powder

♦ ½ tablespoon of paprika

♦ ¼ teaspoon of red pepper flakes

♦ 2 tablespoons / 30ml whipping cream

INSTRUCTIONS:

1. Brown the beef in a pan and drain any grease

2. Add the beef to the slow cooker with the cubed cream cheese, canned tomatoes, chilli powder, paprika, cumin, red pepper flakes, salt, and pepper

3. Stir thoroughly to combine all the Ingredients

4. Add the broth and cream and stir again

5. Cook for 4 hours on a high setting

6. Stir before dishing up

Dinner - Pork Tenderloin (See page 57)

Dessert - Coffee and Raspberry Cream Cheesecake (See page 77)

DAY FIVE

Breakfast - Mexican Casserole Breakfast (See page 37)

Lunch - Instant Steak Fajitas (See page 43)

Dinner – Bolognese Brilliance

Time: 4 hours / Serving 4

Net Carbs: 8g / 0.28oz Fat: 12g / 0.42oz

Protein:25g / 0.88oz Kcal: 251

INGREDIENTS:

- ♦ 1lb / 16oz lean ground beef
- ♦ 1 teaspoon of powdered onion
- ♦ 14.5oz / 411g canned diced tomatoes
- ♦ 3 bay leaves
- ♦ 2 tablespoons of olive oil
- ♦ 1 teaspoon Italian seasoning
- ♦ 8 oz / 235ml tomato sauce
- ♦ Salt and pepper to taste

INSTRUCTIONS:

1. Brown the beef, onion, and Italian seasoning in olive oil

2. Drain the beef and discard any liquid

3. Add the meat and remaining ingredients to the slow cooker and mix thoroughly

4. Cook on a high heat for 4 hours

5. Enjoy

DAY SIX

Breakfast – Zucchini Bread

Time: 3 hours & 10 minutes / Serving 12 slices
Net Carbs: 13.8g / 0.49oz Fat: 15.7g / 0.55oz
Protein: 5g / 0.18oz Kcal: 174

INGREDIENTS:

- 1 cup / 340g of almond flour
- 2 teaspoons of cinnamon
- ½ teaspoon of baking soda
- 3 eggs
- 1 cup / 340g sweetener
- 2 cups / 680g shredded Zucchini
- ½ cup / 170g walnuts chopped
- 1/3 cup / 113g of coconut flour
- 1 ½ teaspoons of baking powder
- ½ teaspoon of salt
- 1/3 cup / 113g of butter
- 2 teaspoons of vanilla

INSTRUCTIONS:

1. Mix the flours, baking powder and soda, cinnamon and salt and put to the side

2. Blend the oil, sugar, eggs, and vanilla until smooth

3. Add the dry to the wet Ingredients

4. Fold in the chopped walnuts and Zucchini

5. Spread batter into the slow cooker

6. Cover and cook for 3 hours on high

7. Cool completely and enjoy

Lunch - Pulled Pork from Mexico (See page 46)

Dinner - Slow Salmon (See page 55)

DAY SEVEN

Breakfast - Baked Breakfast (See page 34)

Lunch - Oodles Zoodles & Meatballs (See page 44)

Dinner – Slow Sausages with Peppers

Time: 3 hours & 15 minutes / Serving 1
Net Carbs: 3g / 0.10oz Fat: 30g / 1.06oz
Protein: 18g / 0.63oz Kcal: 365

INGREDIENTS:

- ♦ 6 x Bratwurst sausages
- ♦ 2 chopped green peppers
- ♦ 1/8 teaspoon of sea salt
- ♦ 2 tablespoon shot sauce
- ♦ 1 chopped onion
- ♦ 2 cups / 1000ml of beef broth
- ♦ ½ teaspoon of black pepper

INSTRUCTIONS:

1. Add all the ingredients to the slow cooker

2. Cook on a low setting for 3 hours

3. Serve and enjoy

Dessert - Pumpkin Bars (See page 75)

DAY EIGHT

Breakfast - Breakfast Casserole (See page 32)

Lunch – Tasty Taco Soup

Time: 4 hours / Serving 8
Net Carbs: 8g / 0.28oz Fat: 21g / 0.74oz
Protein: 26g / 0.92oz Kcal: 340

INGREDIENTS:

- ◆ 2 lbs / 32oz ground beef
- ◆ ½ cup / 170g diced onion
- ◆ ½ teaspoon of ancho chile powder
- ◆ 8oz / 225g block of cream cheese
- ◆ 4 cups / 1000ml beef broth
- ◆ 3 minced cloves of garlic
- ◆ 2 tablespoons of taco seasoning
- ◆ 2 x 10oz/280g Rotel and green chiles
- ◆ ½ cup / 170g of chopped fresh cilantro

INSTRUCTIONS:

1. Crumble and cook the beef, onion, and garlic until brown

2. Transfer to the slow cooker

3. Add seasoning and remaining Ingredients

4. Cook for 4 hours on a low setting

5. Serve with your favourite toppings if desired

Dinner - Beef Short Ribs (See page 58)

Dessert - Lemon and Bursting Lemon Custard Cake (See page 74)

DAY NINE

Breakfast – Stuffed Peppers

Time: 4 hours 10 minutes / Serving 6

Net Carbs: 4.02g / 0.14oz Fat: 15.8g / 0.53oz

Protein: 26g / 0.92oz Kcal: 250

INGREDIENTS:

- ◆ 6 x small red bell peppers
- ◆ 500g / 17.6oz turkey minced
- ◆ 1 teaspoon of powdered chili
- ◆ 1 ½ tablespoons of olive oil
- ◆ 1 cup / 340g cauliflower rice
- ◆ 1 cup / 340g Monterey Cheese shredded
- ◆ 1 teaspoon of powdered garlic
- ◆ 1 cup / 250ml of water

INSTRUCTIONS:

1. Cut the stems from the peppers

2. Scoop out seeds to leave you with a hollow shell (of the peppers)

3. Mix the turkey and spices

4. Stir in the cauliflower rice and olive oil

5. Add the cheese to the mixture and stir well

6. Place a scoop of the mixed ingredients into the pepper shell

7. Pour a cup of water into the bottom of the slow cooker

8. Place the packed peppers into the slow cooker

9. Cook on high for 4 hours

Lunch - Chili Time (See page 48)

Dinner - Picadillo Pot (See page 62)

Dessert - Skinny Mint Chocolate Cake (See page 72)

DAY TEN

Breakfast - Baked Breakfast (See page 34)

Lunch – Instant Meatballs (See page 42)

Dinner – Chicken Stew

Time: 2 hours 10 minutes / Serving 4

Net Carbs: 8.3g / 0.29oz Fat: 26.1g / 0.92oz

Protein: 56.1g / 1.98oz Kcal: 507

INGREDIENTS:

- ♦ 2 cups / 500ml of chicken stock
- ♦ 2 diced celery stalks
- ♦ 28 oz / 795g chicken thighs in 1" pieces
- ♦ 3 minced garlic cloves
- ♦ ½ teaspoon of dried oregano
- ♦ ½ cup /125ml heavy cream
- ♦ Xantham gum, starting with 1/8 of teaspoon until you get the desired thickness
- ♦ 2 peeled carrots diced finely
- ♦ ½ diced onion
- ♦ ½ teaspoon of dried rosemary
- ♦ ¼ teaspoon of dried thyme
- ♦ 1 cup / 340g of fresh spinach
- ♦ Salt and pepper to taste

INSTRUCTIONS:

1. Add the chicken stock, carrots, celery, onion, rosemary, thyme, garlic, oregano and chicken thighs (boneless and skinless) in your slow cooker

2. Cook on high for 2 hours

3. Add salt and pepper to taste

4. Stir in the spinach and cream

5. Thicken by sprinkling gum to create the desired thickness

6. Continue to cook for a further 10 minutes

Dessert - Luscious Lemon Cake (See page 66)

DAY ELEVEN

Breakfast – Egg & Sausage Breakfast

Time: 3 hours 10 minutes / Serving 6 - 8

Net Carbs: 5.39g / 0.19oz Fat: 38.86g / 1.37oz

Protein: 26.13g / 0.92oz Kcal: 484

INGREDIENTS:

- ◆ 1 head of chopped broccoli
- ◆ 1 cup / 340g shredded cheddar cheese
- ◆ ¾ cup / 62.5ml whipping cream
- ◆ ½ teaspoon of salt and pepper
- ◆ 12 oz / 340g sausage links cooked and sliced
- ◆ 10 eggs
- ◆ 2 minced garlic cloves

INSTRUCTIONS:

1. Grease the inside of the slow cooker

2. Layer one half of the broccoli, half the sausage and half the cheese in the slow cooker

3. Whisk the cream, eggs, garlic, salt, and pepper until thoroughly combined then pour over the layers in the slow cooker

4. Cook on high for 2 – 3 hours until brown around the edges and set in the middle

5. Serve and enjoy

Lunch – Baked Loaded Potato Soup (See page 50)

Dinner - Broccoli, Sausage, Cheesy Soup (See page 54)

Dessert - Fingers of Fudge (See page 73)

DAY TWELVE

Breakfast – Ham and Taters

Time: 5 hours / Serving 6

Net Carbs: 17g / 0.60oz Fat: 18g / 0.63oz

Protein: 5g / 0.67oz Kcal: 484

INGREDIENTS:

- ◆ 1lb / 16oz frozen tater tots
- ◆ ½ cup / 170g onion chopped
- ◆ ¾ cup / 255g shredded cheese
- ◆ Salt and Pepper to taste
- ◆ ½ lb / 8oz diced ham
- ◆ ½ cup / 170g green bell pepper diced
- ◆ ½ cup / 125ml milk

INSTRUCTIONS:

1. Grease the inside of slow cooker

2. Layer the ingredients in the slow cooker tater tots, chopped onions, ham, bell pepper, cheese, repeat these layers two more times end with the cheese

3. Combine the milk and eggs and mix well, add salt and pepper to taste

4. Pour the egg over the ingredients in the slow cooker and cook on low for 8 hours

Lunch – Stuffed Cabbage Rolls (See page 49)

Dinner - Masala Chicken (See page 61)

Dessert – Rich Rice Pudding (See page 79)

DAY THIRTEEN

Breakfast – Overnight Apple and Cinnamon Oats

Time: 5 hours 15 minutes / Serving 8

Net Carbs: 32g / 1.13oz Fat: 12g / 0.42oz

Protein: 5g / 0.18oz Kcal: 241

INGREDIENTS:

- ◆ 1 cup / 340g oats
- ◆ 1 ½ cups / 375ml water
- ◆ 2 tablespoons of brown sugar
- ◆ 1 teaspoon of cinnamon
- ◆ 1 ½ cups / 375ml coconut milk
- ◆ 2 diced apples peeled and cored
- ◆ 1 tablespoon of coconut oil
- ◆ ¼ teaspoon of sea salt

INSTRUCTION:

1. Spray the slow cooker thoroughly with oil

2. Add the ingredients to the slow cooker and thoroughly mix

3. Cook on low for 5 hours

4. Serve with toppings of your choice if required

Lunch – Instant Steak Fajitas (See page 43)

Dinner - Pork & Rice Chops (See page 63)

Dessert- Peach Cobbler & Crunchy Oaty Top (See page 80)

DAY FOURTEEN

Breakfast – Slow Cooker Cauliflower Hash Brown Casserole

Time: 5 hours 20 minutes / Serving 6
Net Carbs: 15g / 0.53oz Fat: 8g / 0.28oz
Protein: 12g / 0.42oz Kcal: 356

INGREDIENTS:

- ◆ 12 eggs
- ◆ ½ cup / 125g milk
- ◆ 1 tsp / 4g kosher salt
- ◆ ½ tsp / 2g pepper
- ◆ 1 head of cauliflower shredded
- ◆ ½ tsp / 2g dry mustard
- ◆ Small onion
- ◆ 10 oz / 290g breakfast sausages, sliced
- ◆ 8 oz / 230g cheddar cheese, shredded
- ◆ Salt and pepper

INSTRUCTION:

1. Spray a 6-quart slow cooker with a cooking spray of your choice

2. In a small bowl, beat together the eggs, salt, pepper, milk, and dry mustard

3. Place approximately a third of the cauliflower, shredded, in a layer at the bottom of the slow cooker evenly

4. Top the cauliflower with a third of the onion and season with salt and pepper

5. Top the onion with a third of the sausage, evenly pressed down

6. Top this sausage with a layer of cheese, approximately a third

7. Repeat this two more times

8. Pour the egg mixture over the contents of the slow cooker

9. Cook on a low heat for 5-7 hours

10. Make sure the eggs are set and the top is browned off

Lunch – Stuffed Cabbage Rolls (See page 49)

Dinner - Pork Tenderloins (See page 57)

Dessert- Tasty Dark Chocolate Cake (See page 68)

DISCLAIMER

This book contains opinions and ideas of the author and is meant to teach the reader informative and helpful knowledge while due care should be taken by the user in the application of the information provided. The instructions and strategies are possibly not right for every reader and there is no guarantee that they work for everyone. Using this book and implementing the information/recipes therein contained is explicitly your own responsibility and risk. This work with all its contents, does not guarantee correctness, completion, quality or correctness of the provided information. Misinformation or misprints cannot be completely eliminated.

Design: NataliaDesign

DISCLAIMER

Printed in Great Britain
by Amazon

48265211R00066